Female health and safety

A comprehension guide of the processes that occur within your body

Stefania J. Mundy

Declamer

Table of Contents

title

Chapter Four

Biological factors

Sexual well-being

Chapter Five

Wellness in areas other than reproduction

Chapter six

What Exactly Is the Concept of Reproductive Justice?

What Exactly Do We Mean When We Talk About Reproductive and Sexual Health Rights?

What Kinds of Treatments Are Available for People Who Have Hyperprolactinemia?

Introduction

There are a great number of distinct ways in which men's and women's health are different from one another. The World Health Organization (WHO) defines health as "a state of complete physical, mental, and social well-being and not merely the absence of disease or infirmity." One example of population health is the health of women. The WHO describes health as "not merely the absence of disease or infirmity." The term "women's health" is sometimes used interchangeably with "women's reproductive health," but several organizations advocate for a broader definition that refers to the entire health of women and is better phrased as "the health of women." In developing countries, where women already face more problems because their health is affected by both their risks and their experiences, these differences are made worse.

Although women in industrialized countries have closed the gender gap in life expectancy and now live longer than men, in many aspects of health they experience earlier and more severe disease with poorer outcomes. This is despite the fact that women in these countries have narrowed the gender gap in life expectancy. Women's health is influenced not only by their biology but also by conditions such as poverty, employment, and family responsibilities, which is why gender continues to be an important social determinant of health. Men's health is influenced only by their biology. For a very long time, women have been at a disadvantage in many different aspects, such as social and economic power, which restricts their access to the necessities of life, including health care. Also, the worse the health effects are, the worse the level of disadvantage is, especially in developing countries.

When compared to men's health, there are significant disparities in terms of women's reproductive and sexual wellbeing. Even in developed countries, pregnancy and childbirth are linked to significant health risks for women. Globally, maternal mortality accounts for more than a quarter of a million deaths each year. However, there are large disparities in mortality rates between developing and developed nations. Comorbidity from other non-reproductive diseases, such as cardiovascular disease, contributes to the mortality and morbidity of pregnancy, including preeclampsia. Examples of these diseases include cardiovascular disease and diabetes. The transmission of sexually transmitted diseases from a mother to her child can have devastating effects on both the mother and her child. These infections have been linked to outcomes such as stillbirths and neonatal deaths, and pelvic inflammatory disease has been linked to infertility. Infertility can be caused by a number of other things, and women also have trouble getting abortion services, birth control, avoiding unintended pregnancies, and avoiding sexual behavior that does not involve consent.

Chapter One

Definition and scope

The biological, social, and behavioral circumstances that are specific to women provide a context in which women's experiences of health and sickness are distinct from those of men. The biological distinctions range from phenotypic to the biology of individual cells, and each one presents its own set of specific dangers to a person's health. The World Health Organization (WHO) defines health as "a state of complete physical, mental, and social well-being and not just the absence of disease or infirmity."The health of women is an example of population health, which is the state of well-being of a group of people who are different from each other in terms of demographics.

Some have referred to the current state of women's health as "a patchwork quilt with gaps." Despite the fact that many of the concerns surrounding women's health are related to their reproductive health, such as maternal and child health, genital health and breast health, and endocrine (hormonal) health, including menstruation, birth control, and menopause, a broader understanding of women's health that encompasses all aspects of women's health has been urged, and the term "women's health" has been replaced with "the health of women." According to the World Health Organization (WHO), placing an excessive amount of focus on reproductive health has been a major impediment to ensuring that all women have access to high-quality medical care. Conditions such as cardiovascular disease and osteoporosis, which can affect both men and women, are also present in women in a different way than they do in males. Concerns pertaining to women's health also include medical situations in which women face challenges that are not directly related to their biology. These challenges can include gender-specific barriers to receiving medical treatment as well as other socioeconomic factors. Because of the pervasive discrimination that women face around the world, which puts them at a disadvantage, the health of women is a topic of particular concern.

This broader definition is supported by a number of health and medical research advocates, such as the Society for Women's Health Research in the United States. Rather than focusing solely on problems that are unique to human female anatomy, this definition expands its scope to include domains in which biological sex differences between men and women are present. Additionally, women have a greater need for medical treatment and are more likely to utilize the healthcare system than men. Although a portion of this is attributable to the fact that they have requirements pertaining to their reproductive and sexual health, they also have a greater number of chronic non-reproductive health issues, such as cardiovascular disease, cancer, mental illness, diabetes, and osteoporosis. These are some of the reasons why. Another crucial perspective to have is that events that occur during a woman's whole life cycle (or life course), from the time she is in utero until she reaches old age, affect her growth, development, and health. One of the main goals of the World Health Organization is to encourage people to look at health from a "life course" point of view.

Chapter Two

Global perspective

When examined from a global perspective, gender disparities in illness susceptibility, symptom presentation, and treatment response are especially evident in a variety of aspects of healthcare that pertain to health. The majority of the information that is currently available originates from developed countries, yet there are significant disparities between developed and developing countries in terms of the roles that women play and their health. The term "global viewpoint" refers to "the field of There is no correlation between racial background or geographic location and the fact that women have a longer life expectancy than males do and a lower overall mortality rate throughout their lives. Despite this, women have historically had greater rates of mortality than men, mostly due to higher rates of maternal deaths (death in childbirth). As a result of the industrial revolution, the gender gap shrank and even began to reverse itself in many industrialized countries, notably the most advanced ones. Despite these differences, women are more likely to get sick at a younger age, their symptoms tend to be worse, and their survival rate is lower.

In spite of these distinctions, the leading causes of death in the United States are astonishingly comparable for men and women. Heart disease, which is responsible for one-fourth of all deaths, is at the top of the list, followed by cancer, lung disease, and stroke.

When it comes to life expectancy, the childbearing years are where developed and developing countries have some of the most significant variations for women. If a woman makes it through this time period, the differences between the two regions become less pronounced. This is due to the fact that in later life, non-communicable diseases (NCDs) become the primary causes of death in women all over the world. Cardiovascular disease is the leading cause of death in women over the age of 60, accounting for 45% of all deaths in this age group, followed by lung disease (15%) and cancer (15%). These factors place extra strains on the resources available to developing nations. Changing lifestyles, including diet, physical activity, and cultural factors that favor larger body size in women, are contributing to an increasing problem with obesity and diabetes amongst women in these countries, as well as increasing the risks of cardiovascular disease and other noncommunicable diseases. In addition, the number of women in these countries who die from cardiovascular disease and other noncommunicable diseases is on the rise.

Women who are socially ostracized have a higher risk of dying at an earlier age compared to women who are not socially marginalized. Women who struggle with substance abuse, are homeless, work in the sex industry or are incarcerated have much shorter lives than other women. At any age, the likelihood of death for women who belong to these overlapping categories that are stigmatized is around 10 to 13 times higher than the mortality rate for ordinary women of the same age.

Chapter Three

Social and cultural factors

The World Health Organization, amongst other organizations, is one that recognizes the significance of gender as a social factor that can have an effect on an individual's health. As a result, the topic of women's health is situated within a larger body of knowledge. It is important to keep in mind that women's health is influenced not only by their biology but also by their social circumstances, such as their financial situation, the jobs they hold, and the obligations they have to their families. These factors should not be overlooked.

Women have historically been placed at a disadvantage in terms of their economic standing, social authority, and political influence, which in turn has a negative impact on their access to the essentials of life, including medical treatment. In spite of the recent progress that has been made in western nations, women continue to be at a disadvantage in comparison to men. In developing nations, where women generally face a greater number of challenges in life, the health disparity that exists between the sexes is much more pronounced. In addition to the inequality that exists between the sexes, there are still disease processes that are exclusively associated with being a woman. When it comes to both preventing disease and taking care of people who have it, these disease processes are especially hard to deal with.

Women have been subjected to discrimination even after they have been successful in gaining access to medical care, a phenomenon that Iris Young refers to as "internal exclusion." This is in contrast to "external exclusion," which refers to the obstacles in the way of gaining access. This makes it harder to see how unfair things are, and it also hides the complaints of people who are already hurt by power imbalances.

There are also differences in behavior that play a role, such as the fact that women tend to take fewer risks than men do, such as consuming less tobacco, alcohol, and drugs. As a result, women have a lower risk of death from the diseases that are associated with these behaviors, such as lung cancer, tuberculosis, and cirrhosis. One such aspect that puts women in less danger than men is accidents involving motor vehicles. Due to occupational disparities, women have traditionally been at a lower risk of industrial injuries than men. However, this is expected to change, as is the chance of being injured or killed in conflict. In the United States in 2009, these types of injuries were responsible for 3.5% of deaths among females, compared to 6.2% of deaths overall. Women also have a lower incidence of suicide than men.

Women's health service delivery in countries all over the world is shaped by both the social view of health and the recognition that gender is a social determinant of health. Both of these perspectives are interrelated. Women's health services are an example of a women's health approach to service delivery. The Leichhardt Women's Community Health Centre is one of these services. It was the first women's health center in Australia when it opened in 1974.

Chapter Four

Biological factors

Although variations between the sexes have been documented on a range of scales, from the molecular to the behavioral, the factors that especially affect the health of women as opposed to males are most obvious in those that are associated with reproduction. Some of these differences are not immediately obvious and can be challenging to explain. This is in part because it can be challenging to disentangle the effects on one's health that are caused by inherent biological factors from the effects that are caused by the environment in which one lives. It is believed that differences in physiology, perception, and cognition between the sexes are caused by factors such as the complement of women's XX chromosomes, the hormonal environment, as well as sex-specific lifestyles, metabolism, immune system function, and sensitivity to environmental factors. These factors contribute to sex differences in health. Women can have quite different reactions to medications, as well as very different thresholds for diagnostic measures. When extrapolating information gained from biomarkers from one sex to the other, it is important to use caution due to the aforementioned factors. Older women frequently have fewer resources and are at a disadvantage in comparison to men. In addition, they are at risk for dementia and abuse and generally have poor health. Young women and adolescents are also at risk for sexually transmitted infections (STIs), pregnancy, and unsafe abortions.

Wellness in sexuality and reproduction

During their reproductive years (between the ages of 15 and 44), women face many distinct health problems that are related to reproduction and sexuality. These problems are responsible for a third of all health problems that women face during this time period. Unsafe sexual activity is a major risk factor for these problems, particularly in developing countries. The concept of reproductive health encompasses a wide variety of topics, such as the state of health and functionality of the structures and processes that are integral to reproduction, pregnancy, childbirth, and childrearing, as well as antenatal and perinatal care. The reproductive health of women around the world is given a far greater amount of attention than it is in wealthy countries. In addition, infectious disorders like malaria during pregnancy and non-communicable diseases are also major concerns (NCD). In developed countries, many of the challenges that women and girls face in regions with limited resources, such as female genital cutting, are relatively unknown. Also, these areas don't always have access to the diagnostic and clinical tools they need to deal with these problems.

The wellness of the mother

Even in industrialized countries and in spite of progress in both the knowledge and practice of obstetrics, pregnancy still poses significant hazards to the mother's health. It is well acknowledged that maternal mortality is still one of the most pressing issues facing global health and that it serves as a sentinel event for evaluating the efficacy of health care systems. Pregnancy at a young age has a unique set of challenges, regardless of whether the pregnancy was planned or unplanned, whether it occurred within a marriage or union, or outside of either. A young woman's passage into adulthood is put in jeopardy by pregnancy, which brings about significant changes in her life on multiple fronts, including physically, emotionally, socially, and monetarily. The majority of the time, adolescent pregnancy is the result of a lack of options available to the girl or of maltreatment. Child marriage is a major issue all over the world, accounting for 90% of all female births between the ages of 15 and 19.

Complications that can arise during pregnancy

In addition to the potential for a woman's life to be lost during pregnancy and childbirth, the condition can also lead to a number of non-fatal health complications, such as obstetrical fistulae, ectopic pregnancy, preterm labor, gestational diabetes, hyperemesis gravidarum, hypertensive states including preeclampsia, and anemia. All of these conditions can also be fatal. An estimated 9.5

million cases of pregnancy-related illness and 1.4 million near-misses occur on a global scale every year. This is a significant increase from the number of maternal deaths that occur (survival from severe life-threatening complications). Physical, mental, financial, or social issues can manifest as pregnancy-related complications. It is estimated that 10–20 million women will develop a physical or mental disability each year as a result of complications during pregnancy or inadequate care. This number includes both the United States and other countries around the world. As a direct result of this, worldwide organizations have formulated guidelines for obstetric treatment.

Sexual well-being

Contraception

Girls and young women can be protected from the risks of early pregnancy by using contraception, and older women can be protected from the increased risks of having an unintended pregnancy by using contraception. The ability to decide whether and when to become pregnant is essential to a woman's autonomy and well-being. If more people had access to birth control, there would be fewer unintended pregnancies; fewer women would seek abortions, which can be risky; and there would be fewer cases of maternal and newborn morbidity and mortality. Some kinds of barrier contraception, such as condoms, also lower the risk of sexually transmitted infections (STIs) and HIV infection. Access to contraception gives women the ability to make educated decisions about their reproductive and sexual health, which in turn boosts their level of empowerment and improves their educational and professional opportunities as well as their capacity to participate in public life. Access to contraception is one of the most important factors in societal efforts to manage population growth, which has knock-on effects on the economy, the environment, and the development of individual regions. Access to birth control is regarded as one of the 10 most significant advancements made in the field of public health during the 20th century. Because of this, the United Nations sees access to contraception as a basic human right that is important for achieving gender equality and women's empowerment, which saves lives and reduces poverty.

It is imperative that sexually active people of any age, including adolescents, have access to culturally relevant contraceptive information and methods in order to maximize the degree to which women may exercise control over the timing and number of pregnancies they experience. Even in developed countries, cultural and religious traditions can create barriers to accessing contraception and family planning services. This is the case in many parts of the world, where access to these services is extremely difficult or nonexistent.

Abortion

The term "*abortion*" refers to the process of deliberately ending a pregnancy, as opposed to a pregnancy ending on its own (miscarriage). Both abortion and contraception are closely related in terms of women's ability to control and regulate their reproduction. Abortion and contraception are also frequently constrained by the same cultural, religious, legislative, and economic factors. When women do not have easy access to birth control, they often resort to abortion. Therefore, abortion rates can be used to estimate the number of people whose needs for contraception are not being addressed. However, throughout most of history, the available procedures have posed a significant danger to women. Today, this is still the case in parts of the world that are still developing or in places where legal restrictions force women to seek out underground facilities. Access to abortion that is both safe and legal entails an excessive burden on lower socioeconomic groups and on jurisdictions that erect considerable restrictions. These topics have, on numerous occasions, been the focal point of political and feminist campaigns. Within these debates, differing points of view pit health against moral principles.

Infections are spread by sexual contact.

Sexually transmitted infections (STIs) and female genital cutting are both significant challenges that women face in terms of their sexual health (FGC).

Sexually transmitted infections (STIs) are a priority for global health because they can have devastating effects on women and newborns. Transmission of sexually transmitted infections from a mother to her child has been linked to a number of adverse birth outcomes, including stillbirths, neonatal death, low birth weight, preterm, sepsis, pneumonia, newborn conjunctivitis, and congenital malformations. When syphilis is present during pregnancy, more than 300,000 fetal and neonatal deaths occur each year. Also, the risk of death is much higher for 215,000 babies because they were born too early, had a low birth weight, or were born with a disease.

In addition, pelvic inflammatory disease (PID) and consequent infertility in women can be caused by conditions such as chlamydia and gonorrhea, both of which are sexually transmitted diseases. Another significant side effect of certain sexually transmitted infections (STIs), such as genital herpes and syphilis, is that they can multiply the likelihood of contracting HIV by a factor of three and also play a role in the progression of the virus. HIV and AIDS pose a larger threat to the health of the world's women and young girls. In turn, sexually transmitted infections are linked to risky and often nonconsensual sexual behavior.

Female genital mutilation

Female genital mutilation (FGM) is the ritual cutting or removal of some or all of the external female genitalia. It is also known as female genital cutting, female genital mutilation/cutting (FGM/C), and female circumcision. Other names for FGM include female genital cutting, female genital mutilation/cutting (FGM), and female circumcision. There have been instances in which it has been referred to as "female circumcision." However, this word is deceptive because it suggests that it is comparable to the removal of the foreskin from the male penis during circumcision.

As a direct result of this, the term "mutilation" came to be used in order to emphasize the serious nature of the crime and its status as a breach of human rights. Subsequently, the term "cutting" was adopted in order to avoid insulting cultural sensibilities, which would impede conversation for the purpose of effecting change. Some organizations use the term "female genital mutilation/cutting" (FMG/C) to refer to both cutting and mutilation of the female genitalia.

More than 200 million women and girls who are still alive today have been impacted as a result of it. About thirty countries across Africa, the Middle East, and Asia are home to the majority of those who engage in this practice. Female genital cutting (FGC) practice is very contentious and impacts people of a wide range of religious beliefs, nationalities, and socioeconomic backgrounds. The primary grounds that are used to support female genital cutting include that it is better for hygiene, fertility, the preservation of chastity, that it is an important rite of passage, that it makes women more marryable, and that it enhances the sexual pleasure that male partners experience. The variable amount of tissue that is removed during FGC has led the WHO and other organizations to divide the procedure into four distinct kinds. These procedures range from the partial or total removal of the clitoris with or without the prepuce (clitoridectomy) in Type I, to the additional removal of the labia minora, with or without excision of the labia majora (Type II), to the narrowing of the vaginal orifice (introitus) with the creation of a covering seal by suturing the remaining labial tissue over the urethra and introitus, with or without excision of the (infibulation). In this type, a small opening is created so that urine and menstrual blood can be discharged. This type is the most common type. All additional treatments, like piercing, which are usually thought of as small changes, are included in Type 4.

FGC is opposed by a large number of medical and cultural groups on the grounds that it is both unnecessary and dangerous, despite the fact that it is supported by those communities in which it is a traditional practice. Short-term health effects may include hemorrhage, infection, sepsis, and even result in death. Long-term health effects may include dyspareunia, dysmenorrhea, vaginitis, and cystitis. Short-term health effects may also result in death. Furthermore, female genital cutting causes problems during pregnancy, labor, and delivery. In order to open the scarred tissue, reversal (also known as defibrillation) performed by trained individuals may be necessary. Local grassroots groups, as well as national and international groups like the World Health Organization (WHO), the United Nations Children's Fund (UNFPA), and Amnesty International, are against the practice.

Infertility

The inability of a person, animal, or plant to reproduce as a result of natural processes is referred to as infertility. A healthy adult does not typically exist in this state by default, with notable exceptions made for particular eusocial species (mostly haplodiploid insects). Because they have not yet reached puberty, which marks the beginning of the body's capacity for reproduction, a human child or any other young offspring will typically be in this state. Other young offspring may also be in this state.

Infertility is defined as the failure to achieve pregnancy after a period of one year during which a male and female partner have engaged in unprotected and consistent sexual activity. There are several factors that can lead to infertility, and some of these factors can be treated by medical intervention.

Menstrual cycle

The menstrual cycle of a woman, which is the roughly monthly cycle of changes that occur in the reproductive system, can present substantial issues for women who are in the years of their lives when they are having children (the early teens to about 50 years of age). These include the physiological changes that can affect both physical and mental health; the symptoms of ovulation; and the regular shedding of the inner lining of the uterus (endometrium), which is accompanied by vaginal bleeding. Additionally, ovulation can occur at any time during the menstrual cycle (menses or menstruation). For unprepared young women, the onset of menstruation (menarche) can be startling and even misunderstood as a sign of sickness. In terms of their ability to participate in activities and access to menstrual aids like tampons and sanitary pads, menstruation can place unnecessarily heavy burdens on women.

Women's periods This problem is the worst in lower socioeconomic groups, where menstruating women can be a financial burden, and in less developed countries, where a girl's first period might stop her from going to school.

Changes in a woman's body and emotions that come with the end of her menstrual cycle might be just as difficult for her as the transition itself (menopause or climacteric). The cessation of ovulation and menstruation is accompanied by marked changes in hormonal activity, both by the ovary itself (oestrogen and progesterone) and by the pituitary gland. This transition typically takes place gradually towards the end of the fifth decade of life, and is characterized by irregular bleeding. It is typically accompanied by the onset of menopause (follicle stimulating hormone or FSH) and luteinizing hormone or LH). These hormonal changes may be associated with both systemic sensations like hot flashes and local changes to the reproductive tract like reduced vaginal secretions and lubrication. Hot flashes are one example of a systemic sensation that may be associated with these hormonal changes. Although menopause may provide relief from the symptoms of menstruation and the fear of becoming pregnant, it may also be accompanied by emotional and psychological changes that are associated with the symbolism of the loss of fertility and a reminder of aging, as well as the possibility of a loss of desirability. Although menopause is often a physiological process that happens naturally, it is possible for it to happen earlier than normal (a condition known as premature menopause) due to an illness or as a result of medical or surgical intervention. It's possible that the negative effects will be even more severe if menopause arrives earlier than expected.

Chapter Five

Wellness in areas other than reproduction

Women and men experience the same diseases in different ways, particularly cardiovascular disease, cancer, depression, and dementia. Women are also more likely to get urinary tract infections than men are.

Cardiovascular disease

In the United States, cardiovascular disease is the main cause of mortality among women, accounting for thirty percent of all deaths. It is also the major cause of chronic disease among women, impacting over forty percent of them. Women experience the development of the condition at an older age than men do. For instance, the risk of having a stroke is lower for women under the age of 80 compared to the risk for men, while the risk is higher for those over the age of 80. The overall chance of having a stroke throughout a woman's lifetime is higher than that of a man's. Women have a higher risk of cardiovascular disease than men do, particularly if they have diabetes or are smokers. This is also the case for those who have diabetes and smoke. Women and men are different in many ways when it comes to cardiovascular disease, such as risk factors, prevalence, physiology, symptoms, how well they respond to care, and the outcome.

Cancer

Cancer, the second biggest cause of mortality overall and accounting for nearly one quarter of all deaths, poses a risk of death that is approximately equivalent for both men and women. On the other hand, there are big differences between men and women in how often many cancers happen.

Cancer of the breast

Cancer that originates in the breast tissue might be referred to as breast cancer. A lump in the breast, a change in the shape of the breast, dimpling of the skin, fluid coming from the nipple, a newly inverted nipple, or a patch of skin that is red or scaly can all be signs of breast cancer. Other symptoms include a newly inverted nipple. Pain in the bones, shortness of breath, yellowing of the skin, and lymph node swelling are some of the symptoms that may be experienced by people whose disease has progressed to other areas.

Cervical cancer

Cervical cancer that originates in the cervix is referred to as cervical cancer. It is due to the abnormal growth of cells that have the ability to invade or spread to other parts of the body. The cause is the abnormal proliferation of cells. Early on, patients often do not have any symptoms. In later stages, women may have abnormal vaginal bleeding, pelvic pain, or pain when engaging in sexual activity. Even while light bleeding after sexual activity might not be cause for concern, it could point to the presence of cervical cancer.

Cervical cancer is the fourth most common form of cancer among women worldwide, and it is more prevalent among women with lower socioeconomic status. Women in this community have limited access to medical treatment due to the high incidence of child and forced marriages, parity, and polygamy, and are at risk of contracting sexually transmitted infections due to their male partners' many sexual encounters.

Ovarian cancer

Cancer that originates in or on an ovary is referred to as ovarian cancer. It leads to aberrant cell growth, which then has the potential to infiltrate or spread to other organs or regions of the body. When this process first starts, there may be no symptoms at all or simply very vague ones. The progression of the malignancy is accompanied by a worsening of the patient's symptoms. Among these symptoms, you could also have bloating, pelvic pain, stomach swelling, constipation, and loss of appetite. The lining of the belly, lymph nodes, the lungs, and the liver are all typical destinations that the cancer may travel to after it has spread.

Women who have had more ovarian cycles during their lifetime have an increased risk of developing ovarian cancer. This includes women who have never given birth, women who start ovulating at a younger age, and women who achieve menopause at a later age than average. In addition, obesity, hormone replacement therapy after menopause, and fertility drugs are all additional risk factors. Breastfeeding, tubal ligation, and hormonal birth control are all ways to reduce the risk of developing breast cancer. About 10% of breast cancer cases are caused by inherited genes. Women with a mutated version of either the BRCA1 or BRCA2 genes have about a 50% chance of getting the disease.

Wellness of the mind

During their lives, nearly one quarter of all women will struggle with some form of mental illness. Anxiety, depression, and other psychosomatic complaints are more likely to affect women than men. Women have a higher risk than men.

Anaemia

Anemia, often known as anemia, is a blood illness in which the blood is unable to carry as much oxygen as it normally would due to a lower than usual number of red blood cells or a reduction in the amount of hemoglobin. When anemia develops gradually, the symptoms that accompany it are frequently non-specific and include feelings of fatigue, weakness, shortness of breath, headaches, and a diminished capacity for physical activity. Confusion, a sensation that one is about to pass out, loss of consciousness, and an increase in thirst are some of the symptoms that may be present in acute cases of anemia. A large amount of anemia is required before a person will appear significantly pale. Depending on what's causing the underlying problem, you may have some additional symptoms.

Anemia before surgery raises the likelihood that the patient may require a blood transfusion after the procedure. There is a spectrum of severity when it comes to anemia, which can be mild, moderate, or severe.

Anemia is a significant issue affecting women's health all over the world. Women are more likely to be afflicted than men are, with up to 30 percent of women and 42 percent of pregnant women being found to have anemia. There are a number of negative health effects that have been related to anemia, including a poor outcome during pregnancy and diminished cognitive function (decreased concentration and attention). Iron deficiency is the primary factor in the development of anemia.

Chapter six

What Exactly Is the Concept of Reproductive Justice?

You may be familiar with the concept of reproductive rights, but are you familiar with the term reproductive justice? It combines the concepts of *"social justice"* and *"reproductive rights."* All human beings are included in the scope of reproductive justice. It states that you have the right to do the following:

- Take charge of your own body.
- Make the decision to start a family.
- Make the decision to not have any children.
- Determine the means by which you will bear children.
- Take good care of your children in an environment that is both healthy and secure.

Where did this idea originate, if I may ask?

Black women activists developed the framework for "reproductive justice" in 1994 and came up with the name "reproductive justice." They felt like they weren't part of the movement for reproductive rights, and the goal of their group was to show a more complete picture of reproductive freedom.

Access to birth control, for instance, may be within the law and there may be locations where it can be purchased, but not all people have the same level of access to it.

People who are members of marginalized groups, whether due to race, socioeconomic factors, or any number of other factors, may have a more difficult time obtaining any form of birth control that is effective. Therefore, it may be more difficult for them than it is for other people to control whether or not they have children and at what age.

Because of these differences in access, reproductive freedoms are restricted.

These obstructions are possible despite the fact that the laws prohibit them. They can also take place in a variety of other ways, and it's not just about having the option to postpone having children.

People who live in marginalized communities are also sometimes subjected to coercion in the form of pressure to take birth control or to undergo procedures that prevent them from having the children they desire to have. This does not constitute justice or freedom for reproductive purposes.

Comparison of Reproductive Justice and Reproductive Rights

The concept of reproductive rights is included in reproductive justice. On the other hand, this suggests a broader and more complete view of what this means.

The protection of reproductive liberty within the confines of the law is the primary focus of reproductive rights. They have primarily concentrated on the "pro-life" versus the "pro-choice" debate.

The right to sex education and family planning, which includes the right to contraception, are also included in the concept of reproductive justice. People come to realize that just because they have legal rights does not mean that they have equal access or choices. This realization gave rise to the mission.

There are many obstacles in the way of reproductive health care for many people, as well as the right to choose whether or not to have children. It's possible that this is due to laws on the state or federal level, or even other regulations. It is also possible that this is the result of a lack of safety precautions, health insurance, and/or other factors.

Therefore, reproductive justice brings attention to a variety of factors that influence a person's capacity to make decisions regarding the number of children they wish to have and how they will care for them. These include the following:

LGBTQ people face discrimination, stigma, and systemic inequality.

Economics

Status in society, gender, and racial discrimination.

Environment

Where Do Concerns About Reproductive Justice Typically Arise?

You may or may not be familiar with the term "reproductive justice." On the other hand, it is possible that it will be discussed in the news.

For instance, the Dobbs ruling abolished the constitutional right to abortion, shifting the responsibility for regulating abortion access to the states individually. This is a question relating to reproductive rights, which has the potential to impact reproductive justice. Laws that make it more difficult to obtain reproductive health care are more restricting for people who do not have adequate resources.

Even though the reproductive justice movement got its start in the Black community, it's still important for people of other races and in other kinds of settings. Take, for instance:As a result of the Dobbs decision, it is anticipated that more than half of all states will either outright ban abortion or severely restrict access to the procedure. At the present time, there are states that prohibit abortion no matter the circumstances, states that allow abortion in some circumstances, and states that protect your right to access abortion. People living in poverty and women of color in states where abortion is illegal will be hit the hardest by this. When abortion is not available in a secure and legal setting, there is a significantly increased risk of adverse health, social, and economic outcomes. Because of this, the Dobbs decision contributes to the sexism and racism that have been shown to occur when reproductive rights and services are denied.

In one piece of research, researchers investigated how immigration law enforcement affects reproductive justice. The researchers used the data that had already been collected on a Latin American community in Michigan. They wanted to find out if a raid in the community caused any of the women to rethink their decision to start a family. They came to the conclusion that it did. After the operation, there was an increase in the likelihood that women would want to postpone having children. According to the findings of the study, situations that make people anxious or unsure about the future are likely to discourage them from having children, even if they otherwise would have wanted to do so. In this sense, these are questions pertaining to reproductive justice.

In another review, reproductive justice was examined in the context of the COVID-19 pandemic. This research investigated how the pandemic has impacted people's access to reproductive health care, such as birth control. It was found in 24 different studies that measures such as quarantines and social distance made it more difficult to access reproductive healthcare.

People who have disabilities may also have a more difficult time gaining access to reproductive health care or having the freedom to make decisions concerning their bodies. According to the findings of one study, the number of disabled women who have undergone medical procedures that have rendered them sterile has increased. They are also less likely to use birth control methods that can be removed after a certain amount of time has passed but continue to be effective. They suggest that these differences may be the result of discriminatory attitudes and policies that are directed toward people with disabilities who have children.

The advice that pediatricians give to young patients about birth control is also relevant to the topic of reproductive justice. It is common practice for physicians to recommend birth control methods to all adolescents. However, it's possible that these recommendations don't always take into account the priorities and desires that young people have regarding their own bodies.

A framework for reproductive justice also applies to reproductive technologies, which help people become pregnant and have children when they would not have been able to do so otherwise. These assisted reproductive technologies (ART) come at a high cost and are easier to obtain for those who have financial resources than for those who do not. It's possible that members of the LGBTQ community find them harder to access as well.

The issue of reproductive justice can also be related to climate change. For instance, studies have shown that rising temperatures may lead to an increase in the number of babies being born prematurely, which may have implications for the health of the mother as well as the child. A growing number of young people are expressing doubts about whether or not they should start a family as a result of their concerns regarding climate change.

You can see from this that the idea of reproductive justice encompasses a much wider scope than either reproductive health or reproductive rights. It applies to everything that has an impact on an individual's capacity to make decisions about having children (or not having children) and bringing them up in a way that is healthy.

In general, the objective of the reproductive justice movement is to bring together many different groups to discuss a variety of topics that give individuals the freedom to make their own decisions regarding having children and caring for them.

Access to Sexual and Reproductive Health Services as a Human Right

What Exactly Do We Mean When We Talk About Reproductive and Sexual Health Rights?

In a nutshell, these are the fundamental human rights you have regarding the control of your sexual and reproductive health. It depends on the laws in your area whether or not you have protection for these rights.

Advocates for human and reproductive rights have classified reproductive rights into three distinct categories. These rights include the ability to:

Determine whether or not you want to have children and with whom you want them.

They have access to information and services related to their sexual and reproductive health.

Decisions about reproductive and sexual health should be made without regard to discrimination or inequality.

There are many people in the world who do not have full access to reproductive and sexual health rights. This is especially true for girls and women who live in impoverished areas. It's possible that they don't have access to sexuality education, contraception, prenatal care, abortion services, or counseling.

This is typically the result of the beliefs and values held by a community regarding sexuality, particularly the sexuality of women. There is a chance that women in some cultures are put under more pressure to have children.

Reproductive rights that are restricted have long-term repercussions, not only physically but also socially and economically. Women and girls have a higher risk of passing away during pregnancy and childbirth if they do not have access to adequate options or medical care. Because their bodies aren't mature enough to carry a baby, maternal death is the leading cause of death for girls and women ages 15 to 19 all over the world. This is especially true in developing countries.

If you are denied the right to choose when and if you will have sexual encounters, whether or not you will become pregnant, or whether or not you will have children, your educational and professional options may be limited.

When many young women hit puberty, it signals to their societies that they are ready to take on adult responsibilities. They can end up getting married, having children, and quitting school to take care of their families all at the same time. This feedback loop makes it harder for girls to get ahead financially and professionally, which makes them more likely to live in poverty.

When it comes to your reproductive and sexual health, what exactly are your rights?

The Patient Protection and Affordable Care Act (ACA), which was passed into law in the United States in 2010, makes health insurance and certain medical treatments more affordable for a larger number of individuals. Additionally, the Affordable

Care Act (ACA) broadened Medicaid's coverage to include certain low-income individuals, despite the fact that not all states have adopted this provision. Some medical services are covered by all types of health insurance, but you might not be able to get others until you sign up for a specific plan through your employer, your state's health insurance marketplace, or the federal government.

Abortion

The case of Dobbs vs. Jackson Women's Health Organization, which was heard by the Supreme Court of the United States in June 2022, resulted in the court striking down the constitutional right to legal and safe abortion. Since then, there has been a lot of discussion regarding this matter. This decision gives individual governments the power to decide how they will control access to abortion services.

It is anticipated that more than half of all states will either place restrictions on or outright outlaw abortions. In some states, it is already illegal, while in others, it is only allowed under certain conditions, and in still others, it is a protected right.

It's possible that you're curious about whether or not your health insurance covers abortions. It's a tricky situation.

But more than anything, it is determined by the state in which you reside and the company that offers your health insurance.

According to federal law, Medicaid will only pay for an abortion if the patient has been the victim of rape, incest, or is in imminent danger of losing their life. But Medicaid is paid for using money from both the state and the federal government. Therefore, states have the option of using their own Medicaid funds to support abortions in circumstances other than those listed above. There are some states that do not do that, however.

The state in which you reside is also an important factor. If you obtain your health insurance through the Affordable Care Act, a couple of states mandate it to cover elective abortions, but only if no funds from the federal government are used in the procedure. However, the Affordable Care Act plans and the extent to which they cover abortion differ from state to state. In some states, the Affordable Care Act (ACA) and even some private insurance plans are not allowed to cover abortions under any circumstances.

If you have health insurance through your employer, whether or not it covers abortion depends on a number of factors. These factors may include the location of your home, the specifics of your plan, and whether or not your employer is self-insured or purchases insurance on your behalf. Learn more about your coverage by checking both the guidelines of your workplace and your plan.

Some large employers are providing financial assistance to their employees who must go to another state to obtain an abortion that is allowed in that state. But it's not clear how much risk these businesses are taking by acting in this way.
In some states, it is still legal to have an abortion.

The regulation of reproduction

When you see a healthcare practitioner who is part of your health insurance plan's network, the Marketplace will not allow your plan to charge you for birth control or related health care visits. The Affordable Care Act covers all forms of birth control that have been approved by the Food and Drug Administration (FDA).

- Control of birth by imposing barriers
- Hormonal control implants
- Contraception in a time of emergency
- Sterilization through tubal ligation, also known as "getting your tubes tied."

Pregnancy and nursing are two different things.

If you are pregnant or have recently given birth, you have a legal right to receive health insurance. The Health Insurance Marketplace as well as Medicaid will take care of your health care needs throughout your pregnancy and childbirth. Also, all qualified health plans must cover both care for the mother after she gives birth and care for the baby.

There is no cost associated with receiving assistance if you choose to breastfeed your child. Breastfeeding assistance, counseling, and the purchase or rental of a breast pump are all required to be covered by the vast majority of health insurance policies. It's possible that you'll need permission from your physician.

Other services related to sexual health

The Affordable Care Act (ACA) also pays for the following services related to sexual health:

- PrEP is medication for HIV-negative people who are at high risk.
- STI counseling for high-risk people regarding the HPV vaccine

Adults at high risk for syphilis should get screened. You have the freedom under the Affordable Care Act to select any primary care physician who is part of a participating network. You don't need a referral from your primary care doctor to see an OB/GYN.

Obstacles in the Way of Contraceptive Services

Regrettably, there have been stories of insurance companies refusing to provide coverage for birth control for female customers. Before agreeing to pay for their preferred form of birth control, some people demand women to demonstrate that all other methods of pregnancy control have been unsuccessful. Or, it's possible that they won't cover birth control techniques like the birth control patch and the birth control pill because they use different delivery methods but have the same active components. According to the findings of one study that surveyed 20 different insurance companies across five different states, just 12 of them paid the costs associated with the contraceptive ring, and only 10 of them covered all FDA-approved IUDs.

Because of their religious or other beliefs, some pharmacists refuse to fill birth control prescriptions or provide emergency birth control to their customers. This can be frustrating for patients. This is a right afforded to them in certain states. If this happens to you, you will have to go to a different pharmacy to get your birth control.

It's also possible that the birth control options available to you at your doctor's office are limited. In spite of what they may say, you don't have to get a pelvic exam or cervical screening before getting a birth control prescription.

However, in order to have a birth control implant like an IUD, you might have to visit your doctor twice: the first time for a consultation, and the second time to actually get the device inserted into your body. This can all be accomplished in a single trip.

Remember that it is not required for health insurance plans to cover vasectomies for men. This is something that you should keep in mind.

Additionally, some employers, such as religious groups, are exempt from the requirement that their health insurance policies include birth control for their employees. Have a conversation with your employer about the services covered under the plan they provide.

What Kinds of Rights Do Minors Have When It Comes to Sexual and Reproductive Health Services?

It is essential to keep in mind that young people may have different rights in regard to their reproductive and sexual health than adults. It is entirely dependent on the state in which you reside and the laws of that state.

People under the age of 18 are legally permitted to access birth control, pregnancy care, and STI services in many states without the consent of their parents. This is the case for STI services. In certain states, minors can only utilize these services without the approval of their parents if they fall into one of a few defined categories, such as those who are married, pregnant, or already have children. There are a few states that do not have laws that are crystal clear on parental consent. In these situations, physicians have the option of providing young patients with birth control and other sexual health treatments, but they are not required to do so.

Chapter seven

What You Need to Know About the Corpus Luteum

The corpus luteum is a transient but essential organ that develops in one of your ovaries at some point throughout each and every cycle of your menstrual period. It is responsible for producing the hormones (progesterone and relaxin) that are necessary for a healthy pregnancy and labor and delivery. If the egg that is produced by your ovary goes on to become fertilized, the production of progesterone by the corpus luteum will continue for several more weeks. Within a few days, if it is not fertilized, the corpus luteum will stop functioning and begin to wither away. Throughout your reproductive years, you will experience having a corpus luteum hundreds of times. When the corpus luteum acts in an unusual way, it can cause symptoms that are bothersome or even dangerous.

What is the luteal corpus in question?

During the years that you are fertile, a hormone-producing body known as the corpus luteum will manifest itself in one of your ovaries on a regular basis (about once per month). It has a golden body that ranges in size from 3/4 to 2 inches (2 to 5 cm). The corpus luteum is made up of two types of follicular theca cells: follicular granulosa cells and follicular theca cells.

At the beginning of a woman's menstrual cycle, the ovaries produce a number of follicles, each of which contains an egg. This process is known as ovulation (ovum). At approximately the midway point of your cycle, one of the follicles begins to enlarge, and eventually it will release an egg. Following this process, the follicle transforms into the corpus luteum. The cells of this organism are able to convert cholesterol into progesterone. This hormone is absolutely necessary for a healthy pregnancy.

Where exactly may one find the Corpus Luteum?

Your abdominal cavity houses two ovaries, one on each side of your pelvic region. After the ovum is released from the follicle, the corpus luteum will grow in one of the follicles.

Corpus Liturgy Function

In the event that the ovum is not fertilized, the function of the corpus luteum will cease. In the absence of progesterone, the lining of the uterus will shed, which will result in a period.

If the ovum is fertilized, the corpus luteum will do several things that are important for the pregnancy to continue. These include:

Through the production of progesterone, it gets your uterus ready to accept and care for a baby.

It alters the synthesis of hormones by inhibiting activity in the brain and pituitary gland.

It also generates the hormone known as relaxin. Because of this, the joints in your pelvis will become more flexible, which is essential for a vaginal delivery.

These requirements are satisfied throughout the first 12 weeks of pregnancy by the corpus luteum. After that, the placenta is the organ that is responsible for producing progesterone and other hormones. The corpus luteum shrinks and loses its ability to operate with time.

During pregnancy, the corpus luteum contributes to the regulation of blood pressure through its function. Relaxin is a hormone that relaxes blood vessels and keeps blood pressure from rising to dangerous levels. If the corpus luteum is not there, there is a higher chance of getting pre-eclampsia, which is a dangerously high blood pressure illness that can be life-threatening.

Corpus Luteum Progesterone

The corpus luteum's primary output is the hormone known as progesterone. It has multiple effects on the uterus, including the following:

The endometrium, which is the lining of the uterus, changes so that the fertilized egg can implant and grow.

As the baby keeps growing, the uterus gets more blood to make sure it gets enough oxygen and food to meet its needs.

The uterus itself gets larger.

All of these changes are made so that a fertilized egg can implant itself and grow into a healthy person.

In many different ways, progesterone is beneficial to pregnancy. This causes the glands to become stimulated and also alters the pattern of proteins found in the endometrial cells. During the first few weeks of pregnancy, the growth of the embryo is supported by these proteins. Progesterone also relaxes the muscles of the uterus, which are called the myometrium. This keeps the baby from being born too soon.

The luteinizing hormone, also known as LH, and follicle-stimulating hormone (FSH), are both produced and secreted by the hypothalamus in the brain as well as the pituitary gland (FSH). These hormones are responsible for regulating the menstrual cycle and stimulating the ovaries to release an egg and produce estrogen during each cycle that a woman goes through. Progesterone can stop the brain and pituitary gland from making these hormones and from letting them out into the body.

The effects of these conditions on the corpus luteum corpus luteum defect. This condition arises when the organ in question is unable to synthesize progesterone. If adequate levels of this important hormone are not present, the lining of the uterus will not thicken and will not be able to maintain a pregnancy. You can have a hard time getting pregnant and carrying a child to term. In some cases, infertility issues like endometriosis and polycystic ovary syndrome have been linked to an increased risk of corpus luteum defect. Other risk factors include obesity, malnutrition, stress, and excessive exercise (PCOS).

A defect in the luteal phase Sometimes, despite the corpus luteum's best efforts, the uterus will not respond to the progesterone that it produces. This condition, which is referred to as luteal phase deficiency, is one of the most prevalent reasons why a couple is unable to conceive a child. If you have been trying to conceive but have been unsuccessful, you should make an appointment with your primary care physician.

If your doctor suspects that your corpus luteum is the cause of your infertility, they will request laboratory tests to measure your levels of progesterone, follicle-stimulating hormone (FSH), and luteinizing hormone. The results of these tests will indicate whether or not your corpus luteum is the problem (LH). They may also decide to set up an ultrasound to measure the size of the corpus luteum and the thickness of your uterine lining.

Symptoms That Indicate There Is Something Wrong With the Corpus Luteum

After it has served its purpose, the corpus luteum should stop producing eggs and begin to shrink. On the other hand, it can continue to expand instead and get filled with fluid or blood, becoming a cyst. In most cases, a corpus luteum cyst is completely painless and completely harmless. It is possible for it to occur even in the absence of pregnancy.

Sometimes, a corpus luteum cyst does induce symptoms:
discomfort or a feeling of fullness in the lower abdominal region.
Discomfort is experienced when urinating or defecating.
You are experiencing pain on one side of your body.

Discomfort experienced during sexual activity (dyspareunia)

There is a discharge from the uterus that is tinged with blood even when you do not have your period.

Examinations performed on pregnant women frequently reveal the presence of corpus luteum cysts. By the second trimester, they will have disappeared on their own. In the event that you are not pregnant, the duration of a corpus luteum cyst might range anywhere from a few weeks to several months.

A corpus luteum cyst can continue generating progesterone. When the cyst finally goes away, this may continue for a period of up to three months. These cysts have the potential to rupture on occasion, which might result in bleeding within the abdominal cavity (hemoperitoneum). People who use medications that thin the blood are at a greater risk of developing this condition, as well as experiencing its potentially fatal consequences. Seek emergency medical attention if you have any suspicion that you may have a cyst that has ruptured.

The Treatment of Corpus Luteum

Your healthcare provider will treat a corpus luteum cyst only in the event that it is absolutely essential. The vast majority of cysts shrink in size and go away on their own. Your doctor may recommend surgical removal of a cyst if the cyst is large enough to cause difficulties or if it causes a great deal of pain.

There is a possibility that insufficient levels of the hormone progesterone produced by the corpus luteum are inhibiting conception. If your doctor notices this, they may recommend that you take clomiphene citrate or human chorionic gonadotropin (HCG) in order to increase the production of the hormone by your corpus luteum. Taking progesterone by itself is another approach that can be taken.

Maintaining the Well-Being of Your Corpus Luteum

Because a new one forms at the beginning of each menstrual cycle, you don't need to do anything specific to maintain the health of your corpus luteum. Your overall health and reproductive health both benefit from having a diet that is well-balanced and rich in nutrients; getting enough sleep and rest; and being free from stress.

Chapter eight

What You Should Know Regarding the Hymen

Hymens are fragments of tissue that can be found at the opening of the vagina. Numerous individuals are born with a hymen, and this anatomical feature can take on a variety of forms. In point of fact, no two hymens are the same, and the dimensions of a hymen, including its form, size, and thickness, change from person to person.

The following is essential information regarding the hymen:

What Exactly Is a Hymen?

A hymen is a small and thin piece of tissue that is formed during the developmental phase of pregnancy from leftover embryonic tissue. It is located at the opening of your vagina and is known as the hymenal opening. In most cases, the structure of the hymen is ring-shaped at birth. However, the hymen is capable of transforming into other shapes over time.

In spite of the widespread belief that the absence of a hymen is an indication of sexual activity, scientific research has shown that this is not a reliable method for determining whether or not a person has engaged in sexual activity. In point of fact, the hymen is pliable and elastic, and it does not typically obstruct access to the vagina. Because hymens are made of soft tissue, they can easily tear or break when normal things happen to them, like when a tampon is put in.

What Exactly Is the Function of the Hymen?

The hymen, in contrast to other tissues and organs, does not have any functional purpose in the body. There will be no effect on your body, reproductive system, or health as a result of this.

There is a common misconception that hymens serve as a barrier that prevents bacteria and other microscopic foreign things from entering the body. However, there is no evidence in the scientific community to support this claim. There is scant to no evidence that the hymen serves any purpose or provides any benefits to your body in any way. This is particularly true regarding the function of the hymen.

Hymens that are ring-shaped are in the uterus and cover the whole opening to the womb.

Crescentic hymens are shaped like crescent moons and only partially cover the vaginal opening. Crescentic hymens are the most common type.

In most cases, babies are born with hymens that are annular. However, by the time the children are in elementary school, these hymens transform into hymens that are crescentic.

In extremely rare cases, the hymen may cover the entire opening of the vagina for an extended period of time. When this occurs, menstruation and even sexual activity may become difficult.

What Are the Different Types of Hymens?

There are four distinct forms of hymen, which are often referred to as variants or conditions, and you should be aware of all of them. These different forms are:

An imperforate hymen is a somewhat uncommon hymen type that describes a situation in which the hymen does not open , but rather entirely covers the vaginal opening instead. This can result in a stoppage of the flow of menstrual blood and discharges. Even though this form of the hymen can be recognized at birth, it is more commonly diagnosed throughout the teen years. Adolescents may experience a lack of menstrual cycles due to the presence of certain symptoms, which prevent periods from occurring. In addition to this, a person will typically experience pain in their abdomen and pelvis. Frequently, the patient may also experience urinary difficulties, such as the need to urinate frequently and urgently, as well as the sensation that the bladder continues to be full even after it has been empty.

The microperforate hymen is a subtype of the hymen that is identified when the opening of the hymen is significantly smaller than usual. Despite the fact that a microperforated hymen does not prevent menstruation from occurring, the patient may be unable to insert tampons or engage in sexual activity. Teenagers who are unaware that they have a microperforated hymen may find that they are unable to remove a tampon from their bodies once it has been placed.

The term "*cribriform hymen*" refers to a condition in which the hymen contains an abnormally high number of tiny holes. Normal menstruation may happen, but the person won't be able to put in tampons or have sex through the vaginal route.

The septate hymen is a type of hymen that develops when an additional band of tissue forms around the hymen. This hymen type results in two small vaginal openings as opposed to one large opening. The patient is able to have normal menstrual bleeding, but they may be unable to use tampons or have vaginal sexual activity. Similar to a microperforate hymen, if a teen doesn't know they have a septate hymen, they might not be able to take out a tampon once it's been put in.

The treatment for these variants is a simple outpatient operation that can be completed in a short amount of time. The procedure is called a hymenectomy, and it is performed by a gynecologist who will work to remove any excess tissue in order to create a vaginal opening that is the appropriate size. Once the tissue has been removed, there is no chance that it will regrow in its previous location.

This treatment can be carried out either in the doctor's office or in the operating room, and the location chosen will depend on the amount of tissue that needs to be removed as well as the patient's level of comfort. The surgery is uncomplicated and uncomplicated, and there will be very little to no pain experienced during the recuperation phase.

What Occurs When the Hymen Is Ruptured?

It's possible that you won't even be aware that your hymen has ruptured until it's too late. Some people are aware of it right away, while others are not. Your hymen, like many other tissues, is elastic and may be stretched. Nevertheless, it does not typically tear or shatter on the initial impact. Instead, the hymen will break when it wears down to the point where it can no longer hold together.

In the event that this does occur, you will most likely not experience any immediate discomfort. In point of fact, the vast majority of people won't feel a thing when their hymen breaks, although a few of them might suffer some mild discomfort and some light bleeding. In most cases, however, the procedure of breaking the hymen does not result in any pain. People whose hymens break down gradually over the course of their lives and who bleed may think that the bleeding is just a sign of their period.

It is impossible for your hymen to regrow after it has been broken.

How Does One Break Their Hymen?

As was previously indicated, the use of tampons carries with it the risk of rupturing or tearing a hymen. And so can engaging in sexual activity. However, in addition to these regular activities, there are a lot of other things that can cause your hymen to rupture. These are the following:

- Gymnastics
- Commutes on two wheels
- Riding a horse or horses
- Participating in climbing activities on playground equipment such as jungle gyms
- Exercising
- Masturbation
- Pelvic examinations or pap smears.

Hymen Care

If you're concerned about the state of your hymen during puberty, you should know that any problems will most likely become apparent at that time. If there are problems with your hymen, you might find that you are unable to put tampons in or have sexual encounters. Even if you normally get your period, there is a possibility that you won't have one at all. However, this is quite unusual.

You can also be curious about the state of your hymen and whether or not it has been damaged. Examining yourself in front of a mirror is the only way to determine for certain whether or not you still have a hymen. At the very bottom of your vaginal opening, you will notice a small piece of tissue that is your hymen.

If you experience pain, have mild bleeding, or notice that there is excess skin surrounding your vaginal opening, it is possible that your hymen has disappeared. In the event that this does take place, however, there is no reason to be alarmed because it is a natural occurrence and a broken hymen does not pose any health problems.

When hymens break, they can sometimes regress back into the vagina, or they can remain as a little skin flap on the skin.

Chapter nine

What You Should Be Aware Of Concerning Cytolytic Vaginosis

Cytolytic vaginosis, which is also called "lactobacillus overgrowth syndrome" or "Doderlein's cytolysis," is thought to happen when there are too many of a certain type of bacteria in the vagina.

It is natural for your vagina to contain the bacteria, which medical professionals refer to as lactobacilli. It can help prevent you from infections caused by yeast, for example. Some doctors think that if there is too much, you could get cytolytic vaginosis, which causes uncomfortable and sometimes severe symptoms.

Why does one develop cytolytic vaginitis?

Within the realm of medicine, cytolytic vaginosis is considered to be a contentious diagnosis. There are a lot of medical professionals that do not think that this is a valid diagnosis. Some people feel that the disorder is caused by an abnormality in the vaginal pH balance, although others dispute this theory.

The pH level of your vaginal fluid is an important factor in the overall health of your vagina. It is a method for measuring the acidity, which might change depending on your age, nutrition, health conditions, and other aspects of your life. The range of values for pH on the scale is from 0 to 14.

Vaginal pH levels can often fluctuate anywhere from 3.8 to 5. On average, however, when you have cytolytic vaginosis, a change in pH causes a disruption in the natural balance of bacteria that is found in your vagina. Because of this, the number of lactobacilli in your vagina is elevated to an unhealthy level, and the pH of your vagina becomes more acidic. If you have the illness, the pH level of your vaginal fluid could range anywhere from 3.5 to 4.5.

When a patient presents with persistent discharge from the vagina, a variety of antifungals and antibiotics may be prescribed as treatment. This is a common observation made by medical professionals. But these therapies can change the pH of your vagina and cause bacteria to grow too much in your vagina.

In addition to these treatments, cytolytic vaginosis can be brought on by a variety of additional factors. There's a possibility that your body has a sensitivity to specific items. Some examples are:

- Soaps for menstrual pads
- Wipes\sLubricants

What Symptoms Do You Get When You Have Cytolytic Vaginosis?

There is a possibility that the symptoms of this ailment will be similar to those of a yeast infection or bacterial vaginosis. In contrast, the symptoms of cytolytic vaginosis tend to become more severe in the week leading up to a woman's menstruation. This is because during this part of your menstrual cycle, your body has a lot more lactobacilli than usual.

In a similar vein, the negative symptoms of this condition typically start to subside when you start your period. This occurs due to the fact that menstrual blood has a lower pH value, making it less acidic. So, when you get your period, your body's acidity levels will probably go back to normal when you bleed.

You may find that, as a result of this condition,
Itches in your vagina or on your vulva, which is the skin that surrounds your vagina and is located outside of it.
There is a burning sensation in your vulva, which may become more severe whenever you urinate. Sometimes it feels like the burning sensation you get when you urinate when you have an infection in your urinary tract (UTI).
Aching or burning sensations experienced during or after sexual activity, or both.
Your vaginal discharge has become more yellowish or whitish in color. The constancy of this may shift over time.

How can medical professionals make a diagnosis of cytolytic vaginosis?

A pelvic exam is the first step that your doctor will take in determining whether or not you have cytolytic vaginosis. They will collect a sample of the discharge that is coming from your vagina and examine it under a microscope. They will be looking for cellular alterations as well as a high quantity of lactobacilli and a low level of white blood cells. If doctors uncover all of these things, it could indicate that you have a condition called cytolytic vaginosis.

Your vaginal pH will be measured to determine whether or not it falls within the range that is normal for cases of cytolytic vaginosis. Your doctor could give you a Pap smear to find out if you have cytolytic vaginosis.

To prove beyond a reasonable doubt that your symptoms are caused by this common sexually transmitted infection from a parasite, there should be no signs of yeast, bacterial vaginosis, or trichomoniasis.

What Kinds of Treatments Are Available for Cytolytic Vaginosis?

In order to get rid of cytolytic vaginosis, you will need to increase the pH of your vaginal fluid and return the amount of lactobacilli to normal levels. In order to accomplish this goal, your physician may suggest that you undergo treatment with baking soda. It is also important that you don't use any products that trigger your reactions.

Vaginal suppository Baking soda can be used to manufacture a suppository if desired. Baking soda should be placed inside an empty gelatin capsule, which can be obtained from establishments that specialize in the sale of health foods. You should vaginally insert one capsule twice a week for the next two weeks.

Douche. Mix one heaping teaspoon of baking soda with twenty ounces of warm water and allow it to dissolve. For the next seven to fourteen days, use this concoction as a douche.

A douche bag is something that may be purchased at the pharmacy in your town. In the event that you do not wish to manufacture your own, you may simply go to the store and purchase a baking soda douche that is available without a prescription.

Paste.. A paste could be helpful if you experience burning or itching in the area that is located outside of your vagina. A fluid combination can be made by combining baking soda and water in the appropriate proportions. Always keep this on hand and apply it to your skin.

Sitz bath. In a warm bath, combine two to four tablespoons of baking soda with two inches of warm water. Soak in the water for fifteen to twenty minutes, twice a day, or many times a week at the most. After the first treatment, do this procedure once or twice a week to make it less likely that you will get cytolytic vaginosis again.

If after two weeks of treatment your symptoms have not improved, you should make another appointment with your primary care physician.

What are Some Ways to Avoid Getting Cytolytic Vaginosis?

- You can lower your chance of getting cytolytic vaginosis by making simple changes to your life, such as:

- You should avoid getting soap anywhere near or on your vagina. Simply wash that area with water or make use of a bar soap that is pH-balanced and odorless.

Because menstrual blood raises vaginal pH, you should change to pads rather than tampons when you are having your period.

- You should avoid using scented vaginal hygiene products such as powders, sprays, pads, toilet paper, and other items.
- Changing out of wet clothes as soon as you can is always recommended. This includes swimwear, workout gear, and any other articles of clothing that may become wet.
- Avoid wearing anything that is too constricting.
- Wear underwear made of cotton when you are awake. If at all feasible, you should go to bed naked.
- If you have cytolytic vaginosis, you shouldn't do anything sexual until your symptoms go away.

Chapter Ten

Following an abortion

If you have recently had an abortion, you may be concerned about how to best take care of yourself now that the procedure is complete. How long it takes to get better after an abortion depends a lot on how far along you were in your pregnancy when the procedure was done.

The following are the two types of abortions:
An abortion is a medical procedure in which the placenta and fetus are surgically removed from the uterus. The placenta is an organ that develops during pregnancy.

You will take medicine to end your pregnancy through medical means. The term "abortion pill" has been used to refer to this on occasion.

In most cases, abortions are risk-free procedures, and there are very few severe dangers involved. But it is common to have some minor side effects, like bleeding and cramping.

Whether you choose to have a medical or surgical abortion, it is likely that you will have some symptoms after the procedure. After having an abortion, your physician will go over some dos and don'ts with you. Follow their directions to the letter. Self-care that is done right can help relieve symptoms and lower the risk of bigger problems.

Recovery following an abortion

After your medical or surgical abortion, you should make plans to rest. If you feel ready, you should be able to return to your regular activities the following day, including your job. But for the first few days, you shouldn't do any physical activity that hurts or is too strenuous.

Do not get behind the wheel for at least 8 hours if your doctor prescribed pain medication for your abortion, especially opioids. If you received intravenous (IV) medicine during the surgery, you should not drive for the entire following day.

Most doctors say that you shouldn't have sexual contact with someone or put anything in your vagina for at least two to three weeks after surgery.

Your doctor may recommend drugs to diminish the amount of bleeding you experience or to lower the likelihood of you contracting an infection. Always make sure to take these medications exactly as directed.

Be careful to attend each of your subsequent appointments as scheduled. If you had an abortion with medicine, your doctor will check you to make sure the procedure went well.

What Kinds of Symptoms Are Usual Following an Abortion?

Both medical and surgical ways to end a pregnancy can cause cramping and bleeding.

Bleeding. After the surgery, you could experience bleeding for up to four weeks. The amount of bleeding that each individual experiences will be different. There is a wide variety of possible intensities for the flow. After a medical abortion, you may have a lot more bleeding than you would normally have during your period.

When you exercise, you may find that you have more blood in your system, whereas at rest you have less. It's common to have some little blood clots that range in color from red to dark purple. When the bleeding finally stops, the discharge may be yellow or brown in color. It is possible for it to smell sour.

It is recommended by the majority of medical professionals that you begin your period by using sanitary pads rather than tampons. Every four to six hours, you will need to replace your pad. After having a surgical abortion, you should wait until your bleeding has stopped before engaging in sexual activity or inserting anything, including a tampon, into your vagina. If you had an abortion with medical help, you should talk to your doctor about when you can start using tampons or menstrual cups again.

Cramps. The duration of cramps is often a few days. To get some relief from the pain, you could try taking up to 800 milligrams of ibuprofen every six hours or up to 1,000 milligrams of acetaminophen every four hours. It's possible that putting a heating pad or a hot water bottle on your stomach will help ease the ache. Getting some rest can also be of assistance. You might also get relief from your symptoms by using essential oils, practicing deep breathing, or giving yourself a self-massage that focuses on your stomach, back, and hips.

Nausea and/or vomiting may occur. In most cases, recovery from these symptoms takes no more than a few days. In the meantime, you may find that sipping ginger ale, peppermint or chamomile tea might help alleviate your feelings of nausea. You could also chew on some candied ginger.

Symptoms related to breasts. After your surgery, it is possible that your breasts will feel sore for up to ten days. Put on a bra that offers adequate support, and if the discomfort persists, reach for over-the-counter pain medication. Putting ice packs on your breasts could also be of some assistance. It is possible that fluid will leak from your breasts as well, but after about a week, they should recover to their natural state.

A short time after an abortion, you may also experience the following frequent symptoms:

- Diarrhea
- Headache
- Dizziness
- Fatigue

As your health improves, you should notice that they disappear more quickly. You can find relief from these symptoms by getting enough rest and, if necessary, by taking over-the-counter drugs.

More recovering, it is ideal to wear underwear and garments that are comfortable and do not fit too tightly. Because taking the abortion pill can cause shivering, you should have a blanket handy.

What Kinds of Complications Are Possible Following an Abortion?

According to recent research, having an abortion is even safer than giving birth. Even though such serious problems are uncommon, they are not impossible. Here are several examples:

After either a medicinal or surgical abortion, there is a remote possibility that the patient will get an infection. In the event that you have a procedure, your physician can prescribe antibiotics for you in order to lower your chance of infection. During your recovery, it is best to refrain from baths, swimming, douching, and intercourse in order to reduce the risk of contracting an infection. When it is safe for you to resume these activities, your doctor will let you know.

An abortion that is not complete occurs when the pregnancy is not entirely eliminated during the procedure. The risk of this happening after a medicinal abortion is higher than it is after a surgical abortion. A medical procedure will be required in order to successfully accomplish the abortion.

Hemorrhage: While some amounts of bleeding are to be expected, really severe bleeding can be life-threatening.

During a surgical abortion, you run the risk of injuring your uterus (womb), bowel, or bladder. Other possible sites of injury include the abdominal cavity. There is a remote possibility that either your cervix or uterus could tear. Abortions performed later in the pregnancy are more likely to result in this complication.

Research shows that most of the time, having an abortion won't make you more likely to have health problems like infertility, breast cancer, or depression in the future.

When to Get in Touch with Your Doctor

Make an appointment with your primary care provider if you begin to experience any of the following symptoms:

- Heavy bleeding that escalates over the course of an hour or requires you to replace your pad more than once every hour.
- Clots in the blood that are the size of a lemon or larger, or that last for two hours or longer.
- Pregnancy symptoms that persist for more than two weeks at a time are
- Symptoms such as lightheadedness or dizziness,
- An aching in the chest or difficulty breathing?
- Leg problems such as pain or edema

If you have an infection, you may have signs like a high temperature, discharge that smells bad, discharge that looks like pus, or pain in your stomach or back.

When will you next start having your period?

It is expected that between 4 and 6 weeks will pass before you experience your first period after having an abortion. But you can get pregnant before your period returns.

There are a variety of methods of contraception that can be started immediately after an abortion, or even on the same day as the procedure. They are as follows:

A vaginal ring, a patch, or a shot of an intrauterine device (IUD)

After having an abortion surgically, you are eligible to get either an IUD or an implant. If you had an abortion through medical means, you are eligible to have an implant when you start taking your first pill.

After the abortion is over, you will be able to acquire an IUD.

If you had an abortion during the second trimester of your pregnancy, you will need to wait until your cervix has returned to its normal size before you may be fitted for a diaphragm or cervical cap. This takes roughly a month to complete.

Your Emotional and Mental State After Having an Abortion

After having an abortion, there is no correct or incorrect way to feel about the experience. There are some women who are relieved, while others may have feelings of sadness. It's possible that you'll experience a variety of feelings all at once. Because you still have pregnancy hormones in your body, this is not an unusual occurrence at all.

Free and anonymous emotional help is made available by groups such as Exhale and All-Options. Talking to a professional counselor, a close friend or family member you can rely on, or even another person could be beneficial.

Tell your doctor if your mood swings are interfering with your daily life or if they won't go away on their own.

What to Anticipate During Your Visit to the Abortion Clinic

In-clinic abortions, commonly referred to as "surgical abortions," are pregnancy termination procedures that take place over the course of a single day. In most cases, the procedure takes place in a doctor's office or in an abortion facility. A clinic abortion is a short surgery that can be done at any time during the first trimester of pregnancy or the early part of the second trimester.

A look at what in-clinic abortion procedures are and what you may expect from the beginning to the end of a visit is provided in the following step-by-step guide.

How Should You Get Ready for an Abortion Done at a Clinic?

If you are considering having an abortion at a clinic, it is imperative that you first learn all of the prerequisites. In many places, before you may receive an abortion, you are required to first get counseling regarding the procedure. In certain places, you will have to wait for a whole day before you can undergo the treatment once you have completed the therapy. Therefore, before you show up at the clinic, it is best to check in with your primary care physician.

It is in your best interest to get some things ready before you go to your appointment. If you have children, you should make arrangements for their care. It's possible that your clinic won't let you bring your kids in. If it is at all possible for you to do so, you should also consider taking some time off from work.

You should probably also have a few things on hand to make you comfortable, including the following: Ibuprofen, provided that your physician has given you the green light to do so.

Your current list of drugs, so that your doctor can keep a record of them.

An extra pair of underwear in case you have a heavy flow after your operation (don't use tampons or a menstrual cup). Pads in case you have a heavy flow after your operation.

The case for contact lenses and spectacles alike It is possible that you will need to remove your contacts before getting therapy.

After you have scheduled an appointment, the next step is to figure out how you will travel to the clinic and back home again. In-clinic abortions typically involve the use of sedatives and pain relievers, both of which have the potential to cause drowsiness in the patient. After everything, you'll need to make arrangements for someone to drive you back home. Bring a photo ID with you to the appointment, as well as your money and something to read or watch while you are recovering. At some medical facilities, the operation will be performed on the same day as your initial appointment. If you are pregnant for more than 14 weeks, you will likely require two to three extra appointments.

What to Expect When You Get to the Abortion Clinic

Checking in and arriving at the clinic are the first steps in the abortion process.

It is possible that you will have to go through a line of anti-abortion protestors in order to enter the abortion clinic when you reach there. In most cases, "clinic escorts" or "patient escorts" will be waiting outside of the clinic for their clients. They are either unpaid volunteers or paid staff members who work in clinics that provide abortion services or family planning services. Their job is to ensure that you are able to enter or leave the clinic in a secure manner from the parking lot or the main entrance of the building. If you are worried about your safety, you can call the clinic ahead of time to find out if they offer escort services.

You may be able to bring a friend or member of your family with you to some clinics to act as a support person. However, it's possible that they won't be able to enter the room where your treatment will take place in the majority of instances.

The employees at the clinic's reception desk will check your documents and ask you to fill out some paperwork before letting you in. This may contain information about your medical history.

Education on health issues and pre-abortion screenings

After you've been checked in, you'll be shown to a room that's all to yourself. Here is where the abortion will happen, as well as the health education test, any medical exams that are needed, and the abortion itself.

After that, you will have a consultation with a health educator or counselor who will talk to you about your choices regarding abortion, the specifics of the process, and other methods of birth control. In addition to that, they will determine your weight and take your pulse. You do not need to disrobe in order to participate in this portion of the visit.

After that, you will have a consultation with an OB/GYN, who is a type of physician that specializes in the care of women's reproductive systems, including abortion. The physician is going to:

Review the past of your medical treatment.

You should get an ultrasound to see how far along your pregnancy is at this point.

The steps involved in an abortion.

If you are less than 12 weeks pregnant, you will be given oral pain medications such as Vicodin (an opioid pain reliever), Valium (for anxiety), and ibuprofen. These medications will be given to you in pill form (non-opioid pain relievers). It could take the medications anywhere from forty-five to sixty minutes to take effect. These medications alleviate pain, discomfort, and any anxiety that you could be experiencing.

You will begin taking a drug called misoprostol between the 12th and 14th weeks of your pregnancy. This makes it easier for your cervix to be dilated since it softens it. It usually takes the medicine about 20 minutes to start having an effect.

If you are pregnant for more than 14 weeks, they will use medication and small dilating sticks called laminaria or Dilapan to soften and dilate your cervix in preparation for delivery. The insertion itself only takes around five to ten minutes, but the sticks have to remain in place for the entire night.

It's possible that this part of the visit will take up to an hour. It is possible that your loved one or friend can accompany you inside the examination room, but this will depend on the clinic's policies.

After you have received the prescriptions, you will either wait in the room where you are staying or in the lobby area. If you are more than 14 weeks pregnant, you may be required to schedule an appointment for the operation the following day and return at that time. If you are younger than 18 weeks pregnant, your physician may decide to do the surgery on the same day. However, this differs for each individual.

What Does the Abortion Procedure Look Like When Performed at a Clinic?

There are a few variations of the abortion procedure that can be performed in a clinic setting. Your doctor or nurse will be able to advise you on the best option for you at this point in your pregnancy, taking into account how far along you are. During this procedure, your doctor will use light suction, various medical tools, and local anesthesia. In addition, you will be given an oral pain reliever that you will take by mouth. The amount of time required will change according to the method of in-clinic abortion that you select.

Among the several types of in-clinic abortions are:

Abortion through suction (also called vacuum aspiration). This method of in-clinic abortion is by far the most common one. If you are fewer than 14 weeks pregnant based on the beginning day of your last menstruation, your physician will probably recommend this to you. It is a quick and risk-free process that typically takes between 5 and 10 minutes to complete. You might get a light, a moderate, or a deep anesthetic to keep you from feeling pain during the procedure.

You are merely mildly drowsy or relaxed when receiving treatment with moderate anesthesia. You are "consciously sedated" when you have moderate anesthesia, which results in a greater sense of relaxation. The more deeply you are put to sleep during a procedure, the less likely it is that you will respond or wake up.

If you are fewer than 12 weeks pregnant, the full appointment could take up to three hours to complete. Your appointment will likely last between 5 and 6 hours if you are between 12 and 16 weeks pregnant.

The process of expanding and contracting (D&E). This technique is more complex and will typically be offered later in the course of your pregnancy (after 14 to 16 weeks). Your cervix (the canal that connects your uterus to your vagina) will be dilated with the help of drugs and instruments during a D&E procedure, and your uterus will be evacuated with the assistance of suction. It takes anywhere from 15 to 45 minutes, on average.

However, because this is a more complex operation, your doctor will give you drugs the night before the actual procedure to help your cervix dilate so that the procedure can be performed successfully. This indicates that a D&E could take up to two days to complete, beginning to end. The initial appointment will involve cervical dilation in order to get the patient ready for the surgery. This takes roughly three hours to complete. On the day of the actual surgery, it could take anywhere between four and six hours to complete.

Regardless of which operation you choose, you will be required to remove your clothes below the waist and put on a hospital gown. Your doctor will give you an injection of local anaesthetic so that you do not feel any pain or discomfort during the procedure. You have the option of undergoing a D&E while under general anesthesia, which will be administered to you in the form of an intravenous (IV) injection in your arm. Soon after that, you will pass out and be unconscious.

Is There Any Pain Involved in the Abortion Process?

If you choose to have an abortion through surgery, you may experience cramping both during and after the procedure. Your cramping could get worse or it could get better. The symptoms can vary greatly from person to person.

Abortions performed with dilation and evacuation may be painful to the patient during the process. The sensation is comparable to cramps but is significantly more intense. You may have cramping in that area after your doctor removes the fetus from your uterus.

After an abortion, you will most likely have more extreme cramping for a period of several hours.

What Kind of After effects Should You Anticipate from an Abortion Done at a Clinic?

In the immediate aftermath of the surgery, you may experience some light bleeding and cramps, and you'll be required to take a few minutes to rest. You will receive a sanitary pad as well as a heating pad from the professionals at the clinic. You can clothe yourself whenever you are able to do so.

Recovery

After you have had some rest, you may be asked to remain in the same room or in a recovery room for a couple of further hours so that your doctor or nurse may verify that the abortion was successful.

The health educator will then schedule a meeting with you to discuss how to properly care for your body and provide you with specific recommendations. In addition to this, they will write you prescriptions for pain medication and antibiotics to stave off any infections that may develop as a result of the injury. Because the medication you receive during the appointment may cause you to feel sleepy afterward, it is essential to make arrangements for someone to drive you home after the operation. If you can't get home on your own, call a taxi or ask at the abortion clinic if a volunteer could help you.

Be sure to rest after you get home. In most cases, the effects of the drug will be gone by the end of the day. After the majority of medical procedures, you will be able to get back to your regular routine within one to two days. Tell your doctor if you experience any adverse effects at all.

The following arc examples of complications that you need to watch out for:

Fever above 100 degrees Fahrenheit or chills

in a state of having lost awareness.

There is pain or cramping in the abdomen that is intolerable.

Way too much blood loss.

Infection

If it's an urgent situation, dial 911 or go to the hospital that's closest to you.

Do You Need to Schedule a Follow-Up Appointment?

In the majority of instances, you will not be required to return for a follow-up appointment. This is the case unless you experience any adverse effects or complications as a result of the procedure. Make an appointment with your primary care physician if you intend to begin using birth control or to get a physical examination in the near future.

What You Need to Know About Medical Abortion (the "Abortion Pill")

A medical abortion, also known as a medication abortion, is the process of terminating an early pregnancy by the use of medications that have been recommended by a medical professional. It's possible that you've overheard someone compare this to "taking an abortion pill," but you should know that this comparison isn't entirely accurate.

Getting an abortion through medical means often entails taking two medications: the first pill is taken orally, and the second pill can be taken orally or vaginally. Those who are less than 11 weeks into their pregnancy are eligible for this option. This means that it can have been up to 11 weeks (or 77 days) since the first day of their most recent period for them to be pregnant. A limited number of medical professionals who perform abortions will only do the procedure up until the ninth week of a pregnancy.

A medical abortion, as contrasted to a surgical abortion, does not require the patient to undergo surgery or be given anesthesia (medicine that makes you unconscious during an operation). Instead, you will take the drugs that induce abortion in a medical facility (such as a doctor's office) or at your own home. You must take your medications exactly as your doctor tells you to, both in terms of when and how much to take.

Where Can You Get an Abortion Through Medical Means?

You might be able to locate a medical professional that performs abortions if you look in the following places, depending on where you live:

- Health clinics serving the community

- Private practices
- Hospitals

Most places that do both medical and surgical abortions also offer services for medical abortions.

There are now telehealth programs that let you talk to a doctor about abortion medicine and get answers to your questions through an online video chat.

Verma says that there is evidence that a medical abortion can be done safely even if a doctor is not actively watching you, as long as you have access to the following:
- Exact and reliable information
- Medications for abortion that are dependable (the drugs mifepristone and misoprostol)
- Help in the event of an extremely unlikely complication.

What does the law say about terminating a pregnancy using medical means?

Abortion performed in a medical setting is governed by the same legal framework as other forms of abortion. The restrictions differ from state to state.

It is mandatory for doctors who perform abortions to comply with the legal requirements of the states in which they are licensed to practice medicine. If they break these laws, they could lose their license and face criminal or civil fines.

According to Elisabeth Smith, director of state policy and advocacy at the Center for Reproductive Rights, the laws that set restrictions against the abortion medications mifepristone and misoprostol have an uneven impact on people of color and people living on low incomes. This is the case even though these laws are intended to protect reproductive rights.

Is it Possible to Purchase Abortion Pills Online?

It is dependent on the location that you live in. Different states have different rules about how you can buy abortion drugs on the internet.

If you live in a state that permits the purchase of abortion pills and related pharmaceuticals over the internet, it is imperative that you do so only from reputable vendors. Here is how to differentiate between genuine vendors and those selling counterfeit goods:

Check with the board of pharmacy in your state. The state oversees the licensing and oversight of pharmacies, including those operating online. Please check out the webpage for the board of pharmacy in your state. According to Mary Ann Kliethermes, PharmD, director of medicine safety and quality at the American Society of Health-System Pharmacists, it can provide you with detailed information on rules, regulations, and any internet pharmacies that have been approved in the state.

Make use of internet pharmacies that have been accredited by the NABP. The National Association of Boards of Pharmacy (NABP) conducts audits of pharmacies that are found on the internet. Those that comply with NABP pharmacy practice standards and federal and state legislation are the ones that gain accreditation from the NABP.

Who Should Not Have an Abortion Performed Medically?

Abortion medicine should not be consumed by pregnant women who have.

- In their pregnancy, they have reached the point of no return.
- Carries the pregnancy in an unnatural location (also called an ectopic pregnancy).

- Has a condition that causes blood clots or a severe form of anemia.

- Has adrenal failure?

- Is using steroids for an extended period of time safe?

- Take any medications that might interfere with the process of terminating the pregnancy.

- Has an intrauterine device, often known as an IUD; in this case, a medical professional would need to remove it first.

- Is hypersensitive to the drugs used to induce abortions.

- Can't get to an emergency room if needed. Cannot schedule a follow-up appointment with the doctor at this time.

If you aren't sure if any of these things apply to you, you must talk to a doctor.

What Steps Are Involved in the Abortion Preparation Process?

Your medical history will be reviewed by a physician in order to determine whether or not a medical abortion would be safe for you to undergo. They should also talk to you about the benefits and drawbacks of the treatment that they are going to perform. You are free to inquire about the process with any queries that come to mind.

If you choose to continue forward with this plan and visit a doctor in person, they will want to make sure that you are pregnant before moving forward. If you are pregnant, they will also determine how many days you have been carrying the child. There is a possibility that you will need to undergo an imaging examination known as an ultrasound. Although not for reasons related to medical care, it is required in several states.

Additionally, the doctor could:

- Perform a test on your blood.

- Make you an offer to get checked for diseases that are transmitted sexually (STDs).

Talk to your doctor about the method of contraception you intend to use following the abortion.

A pregnant individual is required by the laws of some jurisdictions to wait a certain amount of time, which is typically around 24 hours, between receiving counseling from their physician and having an abortion. You may be able to receive an abortion on the same day in some other states.

What Occurs During an Abortion Performed by a Doctor?

Mifepristone is the name of the typical first drug that you will take. This is something that is normally done at the doctor's office, although it is possible that they will let you perform it at home.

Mifepristone prevents the pregnancy from progressing in the womb of the woman taking it. This is accomplished by inhibiting the action of a hormone known as progesterone. In place of mifepristone, your physician might recommend that you take the medication methotrexate. This is a less common practice.

After that, you will wait one to two days at home before administering the customary second drug, which is misoprostol. Your womb will be emptied out as misoprostol causes cramps and bleeding to occur (uterus). If you are between 70 and 77 days into the pregnancy, your doctor will have you take a second dose of the medication four hours after the first dose. This will be done between days 70 and 77 of the pregnancy. Even if you have been pregnant for fewer than 70 days, you may be advised by some medical professionals to take a second dose.

Some medical professionals will have you take misoprostol on its own instead of waiting for mifepristone.

Be absolutely certain that you want to terminate your pregnancy before deciding to go through with the surgery. If you stop taking the abortion medicines before the operation is finished, the unborn child may be at risk of developing severe birth problems while they are still in the womb.

What Kinds of Symptoms Might You Experience After Having a Medical Abortion?

During this phase, you should be ready for some pain, like bleeding, soreness, and cramping in your uterus.

Vaginal bleeding: This is very normal, and it indicates that the drug is doing its job. It is possible for you to experience heavy bleeding, particularly in the first few hours after taking misoprostol. You will almost certainly observe clots, and there is a possibility that you will see some pregnancy tissue (particularly if you are more than 8 or 10 weeks pregnant). When this tissue finally leaves your womb, you should notice a decrease in the amount of bleeding you experience. It is possible that the bleeding will continue for several weeks, although after a few days it should become less heavy than a period.

If you go through two menstrual pads in an hour for a period of two hours straight and you are still bleeding, you should call your doctor or see an abortion clinic. You should also make an appointment with your primary care doctor if you don't have any vaginal bleeding after taking the medicines. This could mean that the medicines aren't doing what they're supposed to.

Discomfort and muscle cramps: After taking misoprostol, it is not uncommon to have cramping and pain in the stomach, either minor or severe. Once all of the baby tissue is out of your uterus, the pain will usually start to go away.

You could try taking some ibuprofen to help ease the discomfort, unless your doctor has advised you against doing so due to your health. When necessary, certain physicians will prescribe stronger pain medications. You might also find some relief by placing a heating pad on your stomach. However, you should make sure that the pad is not too hot to touch.

If your pain is severe and the medications or heat are not helping, you should contact your doctor as soon as possible.

A slight temperature, nausea or vomiting, and diarrhea are some of the potential adverse effects that may be brought about by the use of misoprostol.

It's not unusual for these to go away quickly on their own, without having to go to therapy.

Make an appointment with a medical professional if you have any of the following:

- A temperature greater than 100.4 degrees Celsius.
- A sickness that does not go away after a few hours, such as vomiting or diarrhea.

How Does the Recovery Process Work?

Everyone experiences it in their own unique way. A few days is all that is needed for some folks to go back into their regular routine.

Avoid engaging in activities that are likely to result in discomfort. After having a medical abortion, you shouldn't have sexual activity for one to two weeks, nor should you insert a tampon, douche, or any other object into your vagina. This gives your body a chance to heal and makes it less likely that you will get sick.

During the time that you are recuperating, a wide range of emotions may surface in you. These may include feelings of relief, sadness, stress, or even guilt. Consider having a conversation with a mental health professional in the event that the feelings become powerful or overwhelming (like a therapist or counselor). They offer a variety of approaches that can facilitate the processing of what you are going through and help you feel better.

What Should You Expect at Your Follow-Up Visit to the Doctor?

It is important that you keep this appointment so that your doctor can confirm that you are no longer pregnant. You might go back to the doctor who performed your medical abortion, or you could visit another physician who is located closer to your home.

How Successful Is Abortion Through Medical Means?

Up to 98% of women who are up to 10 weeks pregnant and have undergone the surgery have had successful outcomes. People who are between 10 and 11 weeks old are less likely to benefit from it. Because of this, doctors often tell patients to take a second dose of misoprostol, which can make it work up to 98% as well as the first.

The drug is ineffective for approximately four pregnant people out of every one hundred who use it. If this happens, your doctor may give you the choice of having a surgical abortion or keeping the abortion process going by giving you more pills.

The following are some potential warning signs that your medical abortion was unsuccessful:

After taking the drugs, you will no longer have bleeding from the vaginal area.

Even though the treatment has been over a week ago, you are still having pregnancy symptoms like sore breasts and feeling sick.

You continue to have bleeding for more than two weeks after the procedure.

Following a successful medical abortion, you will not get your period for at least the next six weeks.

If you notice any of these signs, you should talk to your primary care provider.

Chapter eleven

What You Should Be Aware of Concerning Endometrial Hyperplasia

Endometrial hyperplasia is a condition in which the lining of your womb becomes abnormally thick. This can cause complications during pregnancy. This has the potential to develop into uterine cancer in some women. Endometrial hyperplasia is an uncommon condition. About 133 women out of every 100,000 are diagnosed with this condition.

What exactly is hyperplasia of the endometrium?

The endometrium is the tissue that lines the inside of your uterus (womb). Changes take place in your endometrium every time you have your period. The estrogen that is produced by your ovaries causes your endometrium to become more robust. This gets your uterus ready for the possibility of carrying a pregnancy.

Your level of progesterone will rise once an egg has been released from your ovary (a process known as ovulation). Your uterus will be prepared to accept an egg if you take this hormone. If pregnancy doesn't happen, your estrogen and progesterone levels plummet. This ultimately results in the peeling away of the lining (menstruation).

However, if there is an imbalance in your hormones, your endometrium may become thicker and expand at an excessive rate. Hyperplasia of the endometrium describes this aberrant development.

What Varieties of Endometrial Hyperplasia Are There to Choose From?

There are two different kinds of endometrial hyperplasia, each based on how the cells in your endometrium change:

Simple endometrial hyperplasia (without atypia). This type is characterized by the presence of healthy cells that have a low risk of developing into cancer. It's possible that this illness will get better even without treatment.

Atypical endometrial hyperplasia can be either simple or complex. This kind is a precancerous condition that develops as a result of the excessive proliferation of aberrant cells. Without treatment, it could turn into uterine or endometrial cancer.

What are the underlying factors that lead to endometrial hyperplasia?

Endometrial hyperplasia is brought on by an imbalance between estrogen and progesterone levels in the body. Your uterus will not be stimulated to shed its lining if there is an insufficient amount of progesterone (menstruation). Estrogen is responsible for the ongoing thickening of the lining. There is a chance that the cells in the lining will become uneven because of how close they are to each other.

What signs and symptoms are associated with endometrial hyperplasia?

The following are examples of symptoms associated with endometrial hyperplasia:

Heavy menstrual bleeding

Continuation of menstrual bleeding after menopause

menstrual cycles that last less than 21 days.

How Can You Tell If You Have Endometrial Hyperplasia?

In addition to reviewing your past medical records, your physician will perform a physical examination on you. They could inquire about your symptoms as well as your menstrual history, such as the age at which you began menstruating and when you went through menopause.

Because there are many different disorders that might produce bleeding that is not normal, your doctor may do some of the following diagnostic tests:

Ultrasound Your doctor may do a transvaginal ultrasound on you in order to determine whether or not your vaginal lining is thick. They will inject a tiny gadget into your vagina in order to do the procedure. This technology generates photos of your uterus by using sound waves, which are then displayed on a screen. It's possible that you have a condition called endometrial hyperplasia if your endometrium is particularly thick.

Biopsy. A biopsy might also be necessary in this case. The lining of your uterus will have a sample of its tissue removed from it by your doctor. This will be looked at in a lab to find out if it can cause cancer or not.

Hysteroscopy A hysteroscope is a tube that is illuminated, thin, and flexible. It will be utilized by your physician in order to examine the interior of your uterus for any problems. In addition to that, they might carry out procedures such as a biopsy or a dilation and curettage (D&C).

Your cervix, which is the opening of your uterus, will be opened (dilated) by your doctor as part of a procedure known as dilation and curettage. After that, they will scrape the lining of your uterus using a small instrument called a curette in order to remove tissue.

What Kinds of Treatments Are Available for Women Who Have Endometrial Hyperplasia?

Endometrial hyperplasia can be successfully treated in the majority of cases. One of the most frequent treatments is progestin, which is a synthetic form of progesterone.

Your doctor may give you a prescription for progestin in one of the following ways:

Orally through the use of injections
In vaginal cream

You will most likely require treatment for a period of at least six months if you choose to use an intrauterine device (IUD). If you are overweight or were treated with oral progesterone, you are more likely to get sick again, and you may have to go to follow-up appointments every year.

Hysterectomy If you have any of the following problems, your doctor may recommend that you have your uterus taken out (hysterectomy).

Atypical endometrial hyperplasia develops when you are receiving treatment for it.

After a year of treatment, there has been no discernible change.

You experience a recurrence of your ailment, or it gets even worse.

Your bleeding doesn't stop.

You will lose the ability to have children if you have a hysterectomy since it will remove your uterus.

Talk to your primary care doctor about the different treatments that are available to you.

Is There a Way to Reduce Your Chances of Developing Endometrial Hyperplasia?

Endometrial hyperplasia is more likely to happen to you if you have any of the following risk factors:

Menopause transition (perimenopausal) or menopause

A history of cancer in the colon, ovaries, or uterus in one's family

Having never been pregnant before

Obesity

PCOS (polycystic ovary syndrome)

Smoking

Gallbladder disease

Disease of the thyroid

There are various treatments available for breast cancer.

Treatment with hormones

The onset of menstruation at a young age

Menopause begins at an older age.

Is It Possible to Prevent Hyperplasia of the Endometrium?

Endometrial hyperplasia can't be avoided, but the following steps can make it less likely that it will happen:

- Quit smoking.
- Keep your weight at a healthy level.

If you are undergoing hormone replacement therapy, you should also take progesterone in addition to estrogen.

If you want to keep your hormones and menstrual cycle in check, birth control is the way to go.

Endometrial Hyperplasia Can Lead To These Complications

Atypical endometrial hyperplasia has the potential to develop into cancer if it is not treated. Cancer develops in approximately 8% of women who have simple atypical endometrial hyperplasia but do not receive therapy for the condition. About 30% of women who have complicated atypical endometrial hyperplasia will get cancer if they don't get treatment.

Chapter twelve

What exactly is high prolactin levels?

The medical disease known as hyperprolactinemia is characterized by an abnormally high level of prolactin production. One of the hormones that plays a role in the process of lactation in a woman's breasts is called prolactin. Also, research has shown that prolactin is important in a number of ways related to reproduction.

The levels of sex hormones in both men and women can be affected by prolactin's presence in the body. At the base of the brain is an organ about the size of a pea called the pituitary gland. This gland is responsible for the production and release of prolactin. Blood problems could be physiological, which means they are caused by changes in the body; pathological, which means they are caused by another disease; or idiopathic, which means no one knows what is wrong.

What are the Roots of Excessive Prolactin Production?

Hyperprolactinemia can be caused by a number of things, such as tumors, certain drugs prescribed by doctors, and other health problems.

Tumors. On the pituitary gland, a tumor or malignant growth might be referred to as a prolactinoma. It is by far the most prevalent factor in causing this condition. The tumor generates an excessive amount of prolactin. The size of the tumor is going to be directly proportional to the severity of the underlying illness.

The vast majority of the time, these tumors are benign and do not cause malignancy. Macroprolactinomas are the medical term for tumors that are less than one centimeter in size. Macroprolactinomas are the terms used to refer to larger tumors. The bigger the tumor, the more problems it causes, such as headaches and trouble seeing.

Medicine. In addition to tumors, the levels of prolactin in the body can also be increased by the use of certain prescription drugs. These conditions are treated with these medications:

- Unhealthy levels of blood pressure
- The regulation of reproduction
- Menopausal symptoms
- Pain
- Sickness and throwing up.
- Stress, depression, heartburn

Talk to your healthcare provider if you experience hyperprolactinemia while taking medication for any of the conditions described above, including breast cancer. They will either tell you what medicine to take or show you how to do things right.

Additional prerequisites If you have any of the disorders listed below, you also have an increased risk of developing hyperprolactinemia.

Hypothyroidism is a condition in which the thyroid does not make enough thyroid hormones to meet the body's needs.

Pregnancy

A tear or puncture in the chest wall.

Shingles, along with other disorders that have an effect on the chest wall,

Other types of cancer that might manifest in the pituitary gland

Chronic diseases of either the kidneys or the liver

Your physician will also examine you for the symptoms of these disorders while he or she is making a diagnosis. Idiopathic hyperprolactinemia is a form of hyperprolactinemia that occurs when the root cause of the condition is unknown.

Women are more likely to be diagnosed with a prolactinoma than men.

What signs and symptoms are associated with hyperprolactinemia?

The loss of bone density, a decrease in sex drive, and infertility are common signs. In addition to these symptoms, women might also experience the following:

Pain caused by vaginal dryness that occurs during sexual activity

Menstrual difficulties, such as irregular or no periods,

Breast milk production occurs even when the woman is not breastfeeding or pregnant.

The following are some of the symptoms that are experienced by men:

Erectile dysfunction is when a man can't get or keep an erection. This can happen for a number of different reasons.

An increase in the size of the breasts (gynecomastia) There is a loss of muscle mass and thinning hair on the body.

How is hyperprolactinemia identified as a medical condition?

A blood test can reveal high levels of the hormone prolactin that are present in the blood. If your doctor finds that your prolactin levels are too high, they may suggest that you get more tests to find out how much thyroid hormone is in your blood.

In addition, your physician will inquire about the medications you are currently taking as well as whether or not you are pregnant. If they suspect that you have a prolactinoma, they will advise getting an MRI to rule out the possibility. This imaging test makes a picture of the patient's body tissues, so doctors can see if a tumor is growing inside the patient or not.

What Kinds of Treatments Are Available for People Who Have Hyperprolactinemia?

The treatment for hyperprolactinemia is condition-specific and is determined by the underlying reason. Some people have high levels of prolactin, but they do not exhibit any of the symptoms associated with the illness. They do not require medical attention. People who have tumors have the following options available to them:

Prescription medications: Your physician will likely recommend that you take prescription medications that reduce the amount of prolactin found in the blood. The vast majority of drugs work well for the people they are meant for and are well tolerated by the body.

Surgery. If the medications are not helping, your physician may suggest that you have surgery to have the tumor removed.

radiation. Radiation therapy is utilized in the event that neither surgery nor medicinal treatment is successful. The tumor gets smaller as a result.

Problems that can arise as a result of a prolactinoma

If you have hyperprolactinemia because of a tumor, you could have problems like the ones below:

Bone loss. The production of sex hormones like testosterone and estrogen can be inhibited when there is an abnormally high level of the hormone prolactin in the blood. Bone density will diminish if these hormones are not produced in sufficient quantities.

vision loss If the prolactinoma isn't taken care of quickly, the tumor could grow and cause the person to lose their eyesight.

Complications related to the pregnancy If a woman gets a prolactinoma while she is pregnant, she might have trouble seeing and get headaches, among other things.

If you are already pregnant or trying to get pregnant, you should see a doctor as soon as possible if you notice any of the symptoms of the disease.